A Lifetime of Misdiagnosis

One Patient's Journey Through Illness, Discovery and Recovery

EVA CARDOZA KING

www.evacardozaking.com

A Lifetime of Misdiagnosis

DEDICATION

To My Beloved Family, thank you for putting up
with me through the nightmare of my
progressive illnesses.
And to Andrea, how do I thank you for knowing
me, and having faith in my character that I did not
have a stress related illness? When I asked you why
you knew I was really sick you said, "Mama, when I
was growing up you never complained about
anything. I knew that you were really sick and that
something was really wrong." Those words have
stayed with me and helped me heal from a traumatic
illness were doctors shun the patient and people
thought that I was causing it to myself. I cannot
thank you enough.

PREFACE

You may be asking yourself why my illnesses and recovery would be something you need to know about. I am as certain as I can be that what I discovered accidentally during my journey of two and half years of illness does affect you, your loved ones, your family, your friends, and the entire population of modern humans on the planet. I still can't believe as I write this that I'm actually still here to be able to write about it. I hope you find my accidental discovery as profoundly significant as I do.

This is an actual true story about me as I became a patient in a nightmare of an illness, who got worse under medical care and who delved into her illness when doctors were unable to help her. It is based on my personal theory of why I got better when nothing the doctors did for me helped, but it is much more than that.

It is a warning that we are at great risk health wise for lack of an evolutionary hormone. It is simple to correct, but most of our preventive medicine from in utero until death does not address it or test for it.

I sincerely believe that 50-70% of all illnesses in modern life are due to one root cause. I hope my story will help you start to connect the threads and allow you to identify root causes of most illnesses you or your family and friends have. We have the science, but it is not yet in practice as my story will painfully illustrate over a period of 2 ½ years. This story has profound implications for health in modern times.

CHAPTER 1

JUNE 2009

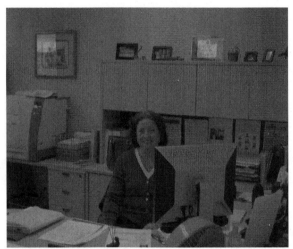

Figure 1 The author just before developing severe Silent Acid Reflux.

It was a Friday night in the middle of June 2009. After work, my husband and I made our way from the San Francisco Bay Area to the foothills of the Sierras in California, as we usually did, to work on getting our retirement home ready. At the age 57, I was close to retirement from my job as an administrator of a fire department.

My husband and I had so much to look forward to. Our eldest daughter and her husband had two beautiful children and lived just down the road from our new retirement home, and we were looking forward to watching our grandchildren grow up.

We had been working on our retirement home for ten years, foregoing vacations and pouring any extra money into the simple and "easy to live in" home, located on a plateau with a beautiful view of the foothills and snow-capped Sierra

Foothills from every room. We built our home together, paid for it as we built it, and named it Casa Dulce Vida after my Hispanic background. We were city people, so we were thrilled to move to the country and still be close to town. In the evenings, we enjoyed the stars for the first time in our lives. My favorite coffee chain was only four miles away and we had the loveliest of neighbors. We had so much to look forward to.

That Saturday, we worked all day on various projects to finish the inside of the house. It was an uneventful day. Just a busy weekend following a busy week as usual.

When I woke up the next morning, I felt as though I had been hit with a hot sledgehammer on the back of my neck and head. In that one waking moment, my life went from utter joy to apprehension and worry. I had severe pain, starting at the back of my neck, moving all the way up the back of my head and radiating through my cheeks and ears.

My first thought was to dismiss the pain as a sore gland or a strained muscle, but I had never felt anything quite like this before. You see, despite my best efforts to stay healthy, i.e. always following the doctors' orders, watching what I ate and avoiding all the things I was told to, I was often unwell growing up and for most of my adult life. I was often sick with a cold or flu, was chronically tired, and I suffered from mild to severe muscle spasms in addition to various other maladies, but this pain felt different. It scared me. And although I tried to ignore it, I did mention it to my husband on our ride back to the Bay Area.

Little did I know that I was to embark on a health-related journey that would fill me with such deep despair, but also a journey of such powerful courage as I would begin my crusade against the modern medical system for knowledge and awareness. This journey would change my entire perspective on the fundamental truths of illness and how 50-70% of all illnesses are due to evolutionary needs that are not being met in our modern society.

CHAPTER 2

JULY 2009

A week went by and it was now July 2009. My apprehension and unrelenting pain continued to grow. I wasn't getting better. If anything, I was getting worse. The pain was horrible across the back of my neck and head.

At the end of a full work week, after not sleeping well, I decided that whatever was going on I knew it wasn't a muscle spasm or a virus. So I decided to go to the doctor to have it checked out. It took another week to get an appointment with my primary physician.

It had been two years since I had seen my primary doctor. I had gone to see her previously after suffering for a year with fatigue and a chronically stuffed-up nose every morning. Upon examining me, she confidently stated, "You have allergies. I'm going to give you a steroid nasal spray. Use it every day." I replied that I had never had allergies before. My doctor of ten years become rather agitated with me, so I set aside my doubts and dutifully agreed to buy the prescription nasal spray as instructed. She restated rather angrily that I had an allergy and to take the nasal steroid spray. As I left her office, I found it odd that she hadn't even looked inside my mouth or checked my throat, as it was a very quick exam. I brushed it off and just was glad to do what I was told.

In any event, I used the nasal spray for a month. It didn't work. So, I decided to just live with the congestion, which luckily seemed to at least lessen after my morning shower. Besides, life was too busy. I just accepted the "allergy" diagnosis and hoped it would eventually get better. Another symptom that I had, which seemed insignificant at the time, was the crackling noises in my throat that occurred in the morning hours as I got ready for work. I chalked that up to allergies as well.

Fast forward to July 2009, and now I had this new severe pain all over my head. The pain was debilitating. I was so anxious. I could hardly wait to see my doctor.

When I was shown to the examination room, the doctor appeared very busy. Probably overworked, I thought as I watched her enter my health data into the computer. After I explained my symptoms, she examined my head, neck and nose and stated, "You have allergies. Are you taking the nasal spray I prescribed?" I said, "No Doctor, the nasal spray didn't work. I used it for a month but it didn't stop the allergies." She replied, "Well, you need to take the nasal spray, as you have an allergy!"

Call it intuition, but I knew that I was being misdiagnosed. Like most patients, I felt it would be disrespectful to disagree with my doctor, so as respectfully as I could, I said, "Doctor, this doesn't feel like an allergy. It's not a stuffed-up nose this time. It's a severe pain in the back of my head and my cheeks, and my ears hurt."

At that point, she became quite upset with me, which is a hard place to be as a patient, especially one who was so desperate to be free of searing pain. She went back to her desk, and wrote a prescription for yet another container of nasal steroid spray. I sat there and said nothing, even though I knew that the diagnosis was incorrect and felt that the examination should have been more thorough. I was intimidated by her professional status. She was a doctor. With years of school and knowledge, she knew more than I did.

As I left her office, I knew in the pit of my stomach I was in deep trouble. I still had no idea what was wrong with me. Having no better plan, I bought the nasal spray and gave it yet another try for a week.

It was a week of pure hell. The amount pain compounded and I went from bad to worse. I hardly slept at night, but still, I found a way to go to work every day and hide the pain that I was experiencing.

Then, one night I looked at my throat in a mirror. It felt rough and it was covered - right up to my molars - with white mucus. I swabbed the back of my throat with a Q-tip to see whether the white coating would come off. It didn't. I gargled with warm salt water. The mucus remained. At that point, I was losing my voice periodically and felt as though I might be developing asthma. In addition, I felt for the first time, that I had been brushed off by my doctor. And that left me in a quiet panic.

CHAPTER 3

AUGUST 2009

It was now August 2009. I felt sure that if I went back to the woman who had been my primary doctor for ten years, she would probably be angry with me, so I decided to try another primary doctor. Someone who would be patient, interested in my symptoms, and curious about figuring out what was really wrong with me. I was desperate for answers and felt being a middle aged women, it warranted a closer look. By then, I had been experiencing pain for about six weeks. The doctor I selected to see just so happened to work down the hall from my first primary doctor. At the time, it didn't occur to me that this might be a problem.

When the new doctor entered the examination room, I felt instantly that she was already upset with me. I pretended not to notice and explained as calmly as I could that I had severe head, cheek, ear and nose pain. Without examining me, she said angrily, "You were told by your previous doctor that you have an allergy and to take the nasal spray!"

I was totally shocked. I replied respectfully that the nasal spray wasn't working. Obviously agitated, she responded, "Like you were told, take the nasal spray. Take it for two months, and if the pain doesn't go away, then there is nothing more we can do for you!" And abruptly left the room.

I was speechless and frightened. Had I fallen into the twilight zone? I was in serious trouble, like life-and-death trouble, and didn't understand how that had come to be. I had been with this medical provider and hospital for 30 years. Basically, I paid a premium each month for thirty years. I couldn't help wondering what had happened to all the Dr. Marcus Welbys of the world. I simply didn't know what to do next.

Another thing I couldn't understand is why both doctors treated me with such hostility. I began to feel ashamed. Ashamed of being sick and ashamed of being dismissed by my doctors.

The undiagnosed illness was threatening to derail my life. And yet, I told myself that I had to hold on – just one more year until my retirement. I didn't want my coworkers to start worrying about me. I dreaded the thought of my illness impacting anyone's life at home or at work. So I managed somehow to keep it to myself as much as possible. This was a difficult task, considering the substantial pain that I was in while simultaneously feeling scared, alone and discouraged.

CHAPTER 4

AUGUST 2009

I was definitely not fine. By August, my nose and nasal passages hurt so bad that I was barely able to sleep. The white mucus on my throat was now creeping into my mouth. And I was losing my voice all day long and it felt as though I had asthma. It had become hard to breathe.

Trying to figure out a way that I could obtain a correct diagnosis, I decided to use the doctor's "allergy" diagnosis to get a third opinion. In an email to the new primary doctor, the one who had obviously forgotten her oath of medical practice, I documented my repeated symptoms and the fact that the nasal spray just wasn't relieving the severe pain throughout my entire head. And since she had diagnosed me with allergies, I requested if I might have a referral to see an allergy specialist? Much to my surprise, she granted my request without comment.

What a feeling of relief!! But I had two more weeks of pain and fear to bear while waiting to see the allergy specialist.

In mid-August, I met with the allergy specialist. I tried to describe calmly my pain of the past two months and the burden of not knowing what was going on. "Doctor," I said, "there is something really wrong with me."

When I finished, he quietly asked me to get up on the examination table. I was shaking from the experience of not being heard by other doctors. The specialist examined me for about one minute. At least he actually looked at the inside of my mouth. "Eva," he said, "you don't have allergies. You have silent acid reflux." Then he handed me a brochure and said, "Read this and follow me."

It was all so quick. Wait, what? I was having trouble wrapping my mind around the words "silent acid reflux." I followed the allergist to his office. He proceeded to begin typing on his computer. He turned around and asked me a series of questions. He didn't make any other conversation. He didn't explain what silent acid reflux was. I couldn't quite grasp the diagnosis, but at least I had one. I was anxious to hear what was next. He asked in rapid succession:

Q: "Have you had a throat culture done yet?"

A: "No," I replied.

He typed. "Well you're getting one today, he said.

Q; "Have you had any allergy tests done?"

A: "No," I said.

He typed. "You're getting one today," he said.

Q: "Have you had your sinuses scanned?"

A: "No," I said.

He typed. "Well, you're getting it done today," he said.

And with that he walked me to the nurse, asked her to swab my throat and to provide the laboratory work slips for me to have a full allergy test and a sinus scan done. As he left, I asked, "Doctor, will I be coming back to see you?" He replied, "No, you will be going back to your primary."

Okay, I thought. Well, at least I had a different and hopefully the correct diagnosis. I rushed through the hospital, getting my comprehensive allergy lab work and sinus scan right then and there. At least things were moving in a positive direction. I just wanted relief from the pain.

The pamphlet the specialist gave me said that silent acid reflux is similar to gastroesophageal reflux disease (GERD), which causes heartburn, except that silent reflux manifests in the throat. I could hardly believe it could cause so much pain. But at least I had hope, because I had a diagnosis, and I was so grateful to know I was not a crazy person.

The tests came back: zero allergies, zero nasal issues. My nasal passages were clean as a whistle. Contrary to the first two diagnoses by primary care doctors, I had NO allergies. Zip. This I knew the whole time, but I was at a loss as to how my first two primaries could tell me otherwise.

To this day I cannot figure out why the first two doctors would continue to insist that I use steroid nasal spray even though it wasn't working. That lack of caring really disturbed me.

How can a doctor tell a patient that if a prescription doesn't work, "there is nothing more we can do for you"? With time, I realized that the Allergy Specialist, without saying it out loud, had in fact recognized that I had primary doctors who needed concrete proof that I did not have allergies so that I would not continue to go through the revolving doors of an "allergy" misdiagnosis. The tests that he ran on me closed the door on allergies being my diagnosis. He had effectively fixed the nightmare for me of being sent down the wrong path by primary doctors. In any case, I had more important things on my mind: finding a way to stop the head, throat, and ear and neck pain.

What next?

I couldn't go back to my second primary-care doctor. It's impossible to go back to someone who really doesn't want to take care of you. So I decided to stay at the facility the allergist worked at, and online picked yet another unknown primary-care doctor. It was a crap shoot, but it was all I could do. I had always trusted my doctors, but I was feeling that something had changed. Was it the system or my age or the fact that I was a woman? Or maybe a combination of all three things? Or was it that this is what medicine had evolved to – get patients in and out as quickly as possible, keep collecting their premiums month after month, and hope they don't return? Do doctors receive incentives for keeping you spinning in the twilight zone of no referrals to specialists? Are doctors caring for the patient or are they worried about the bottom line?

Aside from the ethics involved in medicine today, little did I know that I would someday come to view the progression of illness from a different perspective and that the cause of my illness impacted everyone on the planet, but I wasn't there yet. I was still hoping the "cure" was within reach. I just had to find the right doctor to get me on the path to feeling better.

CHAPTER 5

SEPTEMBER 2009

As I prepared to meet my third primary doctor, I was buoyed by the fact that I had a diagnosis of "silent acid reflux." And I was trying to give doctors the benefit of all my nagging doubts.

My third new primary-care doctor was a super-nice person – a breath of fresh air. She was approachable. And although I was still in pain, I at least felt better because she seemed to care and I had a diagnosis of "silent acid reflux." Little did I know that I would be forced to become an expert on my illness.

My new doctor said that she was going to treat me for H-Pylori, which I later learned is a type of bacteria in the stomach that can cause a variety of problems, including ulcers. She said she was going to put me on two antibiotics for two weeks. I was visibly relieved to hear it was that simple. I was so happy. I would have said yes to anything at that moment.

However, when I began to take the antibiotics, I began to burn even more severely in my head and throat, and the pain in the back of my head, neck, ears, cheeks and nose got worse every day. I took the medicine, but at great expense. I called the doctor to tell her the pain was unbearable. She begged me to finish it. I complied but at great cost. I was more afraid than ever. I was in a crisis, and my doctors didn't get it. Why were the antibiotics making me worse instead of better?

When I went back to see my new primary doctor, I told her I was worse. She then prescribed drugs known as proton pump inhibitors (PPIs), which reduce the amount of acid made by glands in the stomach. The first PPI didn't work. The doctor then moved me to a stronger PPI, but they weren't working for me. I was becoming worse.

PPIs are commonly prescribed for patients with symptoms of GERD, or acid reflux. On the internet, I learned that they are not supposed to be taken longer than a couple of weeks. The literature indicated that PPIs disrupt the breakdown and uptake of nutrition into the cells, and the microbiome of the gut is affected severely, as is the case with antibiotics. So I knew from research that I was heading down a dangerous path.

This frightened me, but the doctors had offered no other choices in spite of the fact that nothing they prescribed seemed to be working. None of them had time to talk to me. Every visit was quick. I received little information, in spite of asking lots of questions. Their response was simply: "Take this pill."

Although I tried to maintain my daily schedule, I was in constant pain, gripped with fear, and filled with shame for being so sick that nothing worked for me. The best that I can describe my throat is to compare it to putting your hand over a fire and leaving it there. The mental anguish only added to my despair. I think this is one of the tragedies of severe pain: it disrupts one's life, no matter how hard one tries to stay in control. The result is a steady spiral downward. Sometimes I wished that I could exit my body to escape.

With no help available from the professionals, I started doing online research trying to find the cause. Finally, my primary doctor told me she was referring me to a gastroenterologist (GI).

CHAPTER 6

OCTOBER 2009

During my first visit with the GI specialist, he told me he was going to send me to an ear, nose and throat (ENT) specialist, who would scope my throat to see its condition. That meant another anxiety-ridden period of waiting. The ENT doctor inserted a tube down my nose to examine my throat. The verdict was that I had a very bad looking throat, but she wasn't really able to answer most of my questions. The GI, she said, would be directing my treatment. I asked the ENT to tell me exactly what my diagnosis was. She said, "You have laryngopharyngeal reflux." I asked her if she would write that down, so I could see how it was spelled. The allergy specialist had called it "silent acid reflux". Laryngopharyngeal reflux was a new term I had never heard before. I detected a slight air of impatience, but she did as I asked and wrote "laryngopharyngeal reflux" on a writing tablet with her name printed on the corner. Never did I think that I would need that piece of paper someday to prove that laryngopharyngeal reflux – otherwise known as silent acid reflux, or burning throat – was the diagnosis I was given.

As we parted, I gathered up my purse and stood soberly beside the door. I was in a quiet cold sweat realizing I was in trouble with this serious health issue. "Try to relax," she advised, leaning close to me. "LPR is thought to be caused by stress."

I was stunned. The implication was that, after four months of constant burning, stress was causing my trouble and the implication was that I had the ability to control it. It was demoralizing and frightening to hear it coming from one of my doctors.

The reader may be asking why this illness of LPR requires two specialists. LPR requires an Ear Nose and Throat (ENT) specialist to report visual findings of the throat to the Gastroenterologist (GI), who is the specialist who decides what to do for the illness. The Gastroenterologist exams the esophageal tube and stomach, but not the throat.

At home I turned on my computer and began inserting "laryngopharyngeal reflux" into the web query line. The articles that came up gave me some insight into what I was in for. For the next two years, I joined online support groups and read every scientific and medical article that might provide a clue as to the cause of my illness, and what might be done about it. I came across articles by doctors who at least recognized how severely the disorder can impact one's life, and who even recommended special diets, but nothing worked for me. In fact, my personal research indicated that there were no real answers worldwide.

On my next visit with the GI – again, a brief and impersonal one – he scheduled an esophageal scope. This was a painless procedure because I was sedated and didn't wake up until it was over. When I came to, the doctor leaned over my gurney. "You look good," he said. "Your GI tract is in good shape." Less than a week later, I met with him for the third time. He said he was prescribing a different PPI. I began taking the new PPI, but did not improve.

I was becoming privately despondent, but I tried to keep this to myself and not let anyone know, except my doctors, how sick I was. I just kept taking the new proton pump inhibitor, never improving. I saw the ENT and the GI every two weeks. My dose of the PPI was slowly increased from November through December 2009. In January 2010, six months from my retirement date, I was put on the highest PPI dose possible and left on it. I knew this was risky because of the side effects associated with long-term use I read on the web, but I put my trust in my doctor.

By January 2010, my legs began to feel like lead weights. For several weeks, I struggled to even walk from the parking lot across the street to my job. I called my GI to tell him what was happening to my legs. "Why are you calling me?" he asked. "Call your primary!"

I was speechless and embarrassed. The information on my prescription of PPIs said to call the doctor right away if you develop symptoms. I didn't bother calling my primary. She was not the one who had prescribed the medication I was taking and I didn't need to get another doctor angry with me. I needed doctors to help me figure out why my health was getting worse.

In early February 2010, I felt really terrible – weak and just not able to function properly. When I went to work one Monday morning, I had a constant cough that I tried to hide by clearing my throat. I shared an office with a coworker and didn't want to disturb her. By one o'clock that afternoon I decided I should try to call for an appointment with the doctor. I hesitated because doctors had no time for me and didn't seem to recognize, even though I told them all the time, that I was getting sicker as time progressed – voice loss, weak leg muscles, a persistent cough, shallow breathing, weak legs and now having trouble breathing.

But I had to hang on. I had another five months before retirement. My husband had retired in December 2008 and was waiting for me so that we could move together to our new home in the foothills of California. I had so much to live for.

When I called an urgent-care clinic on that day in February 2010, I was told that there were no more appointments for the day. Would I like one on Thursday? I said, "No, that's OK, I'll see how I do over the next few days." And I continued with my work at my desk. I was careful to make the call when my coworker was down the hall. I didn't want to look as though I was falling apart, but I was. Two hours later, my coworker said, "Eva, I think you're sick and need to go to the doctor today." I told her that I had been unable to get an appointment. She asked whether I had tried another facility. "No," I replied, "I didn't think about it." When I look back, I realize I was losing my ability to think logically. My coworker urged me to try another hospital. "You have to go to the doctor today!"

Thanks to my observant coworker, Rebecca, I managed to find one open appointment in another city at the end of that same day. I left work at 4 p.m. in a heavy rain. The dark February skies reflected my innermost thoughts. At the hospital, an attendant took my blood pressure. "Oh," she said, "a hundred and eighty-nine! My blood pressure gauge must be broken. I'll get a new one and take your blood pressure again when you're done with the doctor."

I now think that the reading was correct, although I never did go back for a second one. The urgent-care doctor examined me and seemed worried. "Eva, you have pneumonia," she said. "I'm going to put you on antibiotics. You need to come back in two weeks and get examined by your primary to be sure it is gone." I went into the rain and dark night, bought the antibiotic and dragged myself home. It was yet another night without sleep, of feeling totally wiped out and not able to take a full breath.

By coincidence, I had an 8 a.m. appointment with my GI the next morning. When he came into the examination room, he walked in briskly, and as he walked past me toward the computer he said, "There is a thirty percent increase of pneumonia on PPIs." I tried feebly to say "Yes, Doctor, I have just been diagnosed with…"

My voice was barely audible, and I was having trouble getting a breath. Without breaking his thought, the doctor continued, "We're going to have to send you to surgery, but first we have to do a pH study on you." I asked about the surgery. He said he was referring me to a very skilled surgeon for a Nissen fundoplication surgery in a city about an hour away. And with that, he said his goodbyes and left.

Much later I went and researched that statement: "30 % increase" my doctor mentioned.   This is what I found:
http://jama.jamanetwork.com/article.aspx?articleid=183 971

"Conclusion: This study found that acid-suppressive medication use was associated with 30% increased odds of hospital-acquired pneumonia, and this result was significant for proton-pump inhibitor use. These results occur in the context of an increasing body of literature suggesting an association between acid-suppressive medication and pneumonia. Further scrutiny is warranted regarding inpatient prescribing practices of these medications."

My doctor did not explain what a pH study was, or what a Nissen fundoplication was, but like I said, he was a busy doctor. I later learned, through my own research, that the study was a procedure to measure the pH or amount of stomach acid in a patient's esophagus, and that Nissen fundoplication is a procedure in which the upper curve of a patient's stomach is wrapped around the lower esophageal sphincter and sewn into place. This is supposed to strengthen the valve between the stomach and esophagus. I felt comforted by the fact that the GI at least could see I was in trouble, but I knew that being sent to surgery indicated they had run out of options for me.

As I left the examining room, it flashed through my mind that the GI did not tell me to stop taking the PPI acid-blocking medication. I thought that was odd after telling me about the increased risks of developing pneumonia on PPIs, but I was too sick to think more deeply.

I pushed myself back to work two days later and took the antibiotics. But as the days wore on, I wasn't getting better. After I finished the round of antibiotics, I went in to see my new very kind primary doctor, as instructed by the urgent-care clinic physician. When she walked into the room, she was carrying my newest chest x-ray and had worry written across her face. After examining me, she said quietly, "Eva, you still have pneumonia." She paused. "You are very sick. I'm not sure what to do. I think I'll see if your body can get over the pneumonia by itself. I'll check you in a week." My searing throat continued to riddle me with unbearable pain. I was more concerned about that than about the half-breaths of pneumonia.

When I went home, I looked out into the backyard and made a private decision on my own. I would stop taking the PPIs and to my total surprise, the pneumonia lifted within 24 hours. I didn't need a doctor to tell me that. I could feel it.

When I saw my primary a week later, she declared that the pneumonia had cleared up. I didn't mention to either my primary or my GI specialist that I had stopped the PPIs. I was afraid that telling them would elicit anger, as had the steroid nose-spray incident, but I knew from my own research that taking PPIs on a long-term basis was risky. My research on the internet told me that the medication could carry serious side effects, and I had already seen the evidence of that.

The pH study done that spring apparently indicated that my score of 40 was high enough to warrant surgery. What a relief! I was beyond hopeful that finally something would work to stop this searing throat pain.

I met with the surgeon in March 2010. Once again I found another indifferent doctor, who looked at the floor when she talked to me. As she looked at the floor she strongly tried to discourage me from having the Nissen fundoplication surgical procedure. She said it would give me only about a 50/50 chance to get better. With my form of reflux, surgery would not work. I strongly and respectfully advocated for myself, explaining how hard it was as a patient to be constantly brushed off. I began to weep. I told her I wanted to try anything to stop the unrelenting pain, and that I had heard she was a very good surgeon. I wanted her to do it. After a lot of back and forth the primary surgeon said she would perform the surgery if a thoracic surgeon, who was part of her team, gave a second opinion that the surgery could help me. I said okay reluctantly. I felt that he too would probably say the surgery wouldn't help me.

A week later, to my surprise and relief, the thoracic surgeon told me that he felt the fundoplication surgery would give me a 90 percent to 95 percent chance of fixing the problem. I was thrilled and full of hope.

The surgery was scheduled for mid-May 2010. I decided to announce my retirement for June 1, 2010. The joy of retirement and our new home was tempered by pain and worry about the outcome of the surgery. I was terrified, but I felt I had no choice but to go forward with surgery.

And then one day at work, something transpired that would eventually help me piece together answers to my illness with time. I realized I hadn't taken my calcium citrate supplement at home that morning. For convenience, I always kept a bottle of calcium tablets at home and at my work desk. I had suffered since the age of about 40 with leg, knee and bone pain. I tried for years to exercise. Exercise never helped my bone pain. So I decided to treat bone pain for 20 years with calcium citrate and it helped! For 20 years my primary doctors had always just handed me a sheet of paper with leg exercises for my bone and muscle pain. The exercises never did help, but the calcium seemed to. This time while at my desk, I took the calcium citrate pill with a glass of water at my work desk and immediately noticed that I had a flare of worse burning in my throat than usual.

Going back to my internet research, I discovered that calcium citrate could aggravate acid reflux, a finding that was confirmed later by my surgeon. So I stopped taking the calcium citrate vitamin two weeks before surgery. I started feeling slightly better for the first time in ten months from stopping the calcium citrate, although I still had throat pain. The surgery was the only option to address the illness.

The final day of work arrived before surgery the next day. I had decided it was time to retire just before surgery as I knew there would be a long recovery and learning to slowly eat again. It was difficult because my future health seemed so uncertain. All that had been a normal life seemed to be changing forever. My new life, retirement and my health hung in the 'balance' of getting well. I said goodbye to my fire administration family and realized how fragile life is. I had a lot to live for and had to try to get better. I was the last to leave that evening because I wanted to savor the last moments in a place that reminded me of a normal life before LPR. I walked out after everyone had left with the flowers and a badge my Chief Jim had given me clutched close in my arms. I was headed into an uncertain future with my health issues.

CHAPTER 7

MAY 17, 2010

On the day of my surgery, I was full of hope but terrified at the same time. This was not my first surgery. I had five surgeries previously. This pending operation seemed like my only chance of getting better, though I knew that there was no guarantee. I gathered all the courage I could muster to proceed.

When the operation was over, my husband and sister were there to greet me. My two surgeons came to my hospital room on their rounds and we all hoped for the best. They told me that for a while, I couldn't lift anything and must stay on a diet of soft, low-acid food, like jello. I could see the concern in their eyes. It was the first time in a long time that I felt that my doctors had really looked at me.

And to my immediate assessment I didn't feel any burning! That is all I could think of. Was it possible that the surgery had worked?! We all agreed that this was good sign (though, I realized many years later, that the acid blocking medications given to me before surgery may have been why I didn't feel burning after surgery) and the lead surgeon actually looked at me as she talked. At that moment, I felt better about everything. That personal touch makes all the difference to a patient. I actually felt joy, even though I was in a great deal of pain from the operation. I was past the worst part. Just getting there was a Mount Everest climb for me.

There was no burning in my throat or pain in the back of my head. I was released from hospital and sent home with medication for pain from the surgery. I had high hopes.

CHAPTER 8

MID-MAY 2010 – DECEMBER 2010

At home, my husband had begun the move to our new home. Everything was packed up and we were selling the house we had lived in for twenty-five years. There were many things to decide – dealing with our realtor, staging the house, and organizing the move. I did as much as I could.

When I arrived home I have several prescription pain medications to take. As I began take these pain medications I began to experience head pain. At the time, I did not realize that the medications were causing the searing throat to get worse and worse as the days passed. It was so depressing. I knew the surgery had failed whether it was the medications or food. It had simply failed. But I found out much later, after researching, was that the pain medications the surgeon prescribed for me were known for exacerbating reflux and that even aspirin will exacerbate reflux. So the medication exacerbated an already failed fundoplication surgery. This was a disaster to have a burning throat that was worse after surgery. For a while, I couldn't swallow regular food – only liquids and liquid food – and I was ravenous after a week. But that was the easy part to deal with. It was the escalating throat burn that was devastating. The lead surgeon was right: the odds had not been in my favor.

When I saw the lead surgeon for my two-week checkup after surgery, I told her my throat was burning. She said she had other appointments and that there was nothing else she could do for me. I had to go back to the GI. I was surprised. I had not realized that if surgery failed there were no other options.

Before I left for our new home, I went to see the ENT doctor the surgeon had recommended. He reviewed my recent medical history with me and examined my throat but said nothing. I asked him what he saw. He said, "You still have laryngopharyngeal reflux."

I could tell it was hard for him to tell me that. I asked what he would do if he had LPR. He said I had to go back to the GI to ask that question; he was just doing the exam and scope of my throat.

I walked out of the hospital determined to find a way to get better. I wrote to my surgeons for four months, and even made a three-and-a-half-hour trip to see the thoracic surgeon. I pleaded with the lead surgeon to re-do the operation. She emailed me that there was nothing more she could do. I was deeply frustrated and angry.

The thoracic surgeon emailed me for several months. I felt that he cared, but even he had no ideas. All I could do was go back to a GI as instructed, but I couldn't make the long trip back and forth to the Bay Area too often because I was too debilitated. After four months, I realized I had to get a doctor in Northern California, closer to our new home.

I was getting worse and worse by the day. There was very little that I could eat – so little that I began to lose weight. I switched from regular water to spring water, hoping the higher pH of 8 would help me get much needed liquid down my throat. At night, I hardly slept because of the pain. I paced the floor at all hours. Meanwhile, family life went on. When friends came by, I felt ashamed to be so sick. I could barely sit still and talk with them, and I'm sure I looked as if I didn't want them there, but that was not the case. I was terrified of what I had and the pain was unbearable.

My youngest daughter returned from law school at the end of August 2010. My husband worked hard to get a pool built and patio and bricks laid in the front driveway and patio cement in the backyard in time for her return. We were so excited to have our youngest back home. It was a massive push to get it all done. Contractors with big, noisy equipment were working on the front and back areas of the grounds. Between the pounding of heavy machinery and my pain, I felt pushed to the brink and getting worse each day.

I was becoming unraveled by seeing my health go from bad to worse. Instead of being able to enjoy the bustle of our new life, I was falling apart, trying to cope quietly.

One morning I received a call from my former Fire Chief calling to ask me how I was. I was in bed, debilitated by pain, and tried to tell him without sounding full of despair, that I was worse and the doctors didn't seem to have an answer. My former Fire Chief said, "Give them hell, Eva. You tell them you want something done." I said okay and decided to make an attempt to set up a primary care doctor in my new area.

In September, about four months after my surgery, I visited my new primary doctor in the region where I lived. I shared with her all the things I had been researching on the condition called LPR, and told her that I wanted to look into a new type of surgery. She told me to stop researching – the new type of surgery would take years to evaluate. I asked her if she would try to find out what alternatives there were for someone with severe LPR. She said she would, but she never did. She was very nice, but obviously very busy.

One day my head and throat pain was so severe, I drove myself to the Emergency Room (ER) of the hospital about one hour away. At the ER window I began to weep. I had reached a point where I could not take the throat pain anymore. After I explained to the ER nurse why I was there, she entered my information in a chart, barely glancing at me. Then the staff put me on a gurney, where I waited for a doctor in a dark corner of the ER. When the doctor finally arrived, I told him about my recent medical history, and that I had lost 30 pounds in two months because I couldn't eat. He was quiet and then left.

To my surprise, the ER doctor came back later and told me that he was ordering Behavioral Science appointments for me. I was devastated. I didn't have the sense to request an ENT. I was by myself and too debilitated to advocate for myself. My condition had deteriorated so severely that I wasn't able to think clearly anymore. I realized they thought that my illness was stress related and somehow I was causing it. They did not think it was a physical illness.

I drove home alone just after midnight and got lost on the unfamiliar freeway, as the highway was closed down for road construction. I went in circles trying to find a way home. And I was both scared at being lost and scared being so alone with unrelenting pain.

In the next few weeks, I felt utterly hopeless. I felt that I would just wither away and die if I didn't stop losing weight. I gave in to the ridiculous Behavioral Science referral. I accepted whatever the doctors wanted to do. I knew they were wrong, but I had no more fight left in me.

I kept several appointments with the Behavioral Science specialists. They asked me in different ways whether I had any stress that could be causing this problem. I said quietly each and every time, "The only stress I have is burning to death. I'm happy, just retired, my daughters are grown, and my husband just built us a beautiful home and pool. I've never been happier." I know I must have looked forlorn. But pain really changes how one looks.

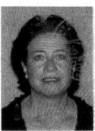

Figure 2 Author just before surgery. Note the sides of the throat are swollen.

In the meantime, I asked my primary doctor to arrange for a new GI for me at the local hospital. (This was not done by the ER doctor even though my records showed I had just had a GI surgery. I, the patient, had to request it.) I discovered that the new GI had been a specialist for 30 years. This made me feel better. Maybe she had seen a case like mine. Maybe someone had an idea how to treat this problem.

My hopes were dashed when she walked into the examination room. She already appeared angry with me. She asked me to explain everything that had occurred with this illness. I did my best, although I could barely talk due to the burn ulcers in my throat. I detected immediately that she didn't believe a word I said.

I told her that my medical record should confirm everything that I told her. She replied that my record did not do so. I had just told her that two ENTs in the Bay Area had diagnosed laryngopharyngeal reflux. She said my record didn't say that. She basically was telling me that everything I said was not on my record. I was dumbfounded. I felt as though I was in another reality – the twilight zone.

I did my best to explain everything in chronological order. With barely controlled anger, she turned her computer monitor around to face me and said, "Look at the screen. It doesn't say that!" I was so shocked, I couldn't focus on the screen. All I could say was, "Doctor, I have tried to describe everything as I remember it and as it happened and what was told to me." "Well," she said, "it doesn't say any of that."

She continued to type on her computer keyboard and then said she would examine me. She was still visibly hostile. Maybe she thought I was a chronic complainer, which I am not. Looking back, I have concluded that somehow I got labeled early on as a stress patient. The doctors, it appeared, had done the surgery and that was probably all they could do. They wanted me to stop coming back to them.

After her physical exam, she saw that I was in pain, especially after touching the sides of my neck. She did call to make an appointment with ENT before she sent me to primary. She did not say a word to me as I left her office, even after I thanked her. Though I'm not sure why I thanked her. Her conduct as a physician was despicable, but I have my dignity and tried to act like I didn't see it. To this day I'm still baffled by why I was treated this way. The only thing I can think of is that they felt my condition was stress related and my records where not fully loaded into the Northern

California facility after my move, so maybe she could not see them. I don't know, but I felt the hostility coming from the GI doctor was unacceptable.

A week later, I was seen by a new ENT. He was a gregarious and warm doctor. I liked him right away. As he scoped my throat, he gasped at its condition. He said it was in extremely bad condition. He said I had numerous burn ulcers on my whole throat and they were raw burns. I wanted to burst into tears, I was so desperate, but at least I knew I wasn't a crazy person. I worried about this condition becoming malignant the more time went on, and my fears increased as he looked farther down at the back of my esophagus. He said he had to do a biopsy immediately as my condition may have progressed to cancer.

I cried quietly and told him to give me just a little bit of time. I shared that at times the severity of my throat made me feel like I had a fever. My throat hurt so much that I couldn't bear the idea of a biopsy. I trembled from pain. I tried to hide the trembling because I was so ashamed by now of being so sick and nothing working on me. Then the ENT told me that there was a separate issue, involving my thyroid. It had a large growth that was pushing my esophagus to the side. He said there was a good chance I had cancer in the thyroid, too, but he emphasized the thyroid and my throat were two separate issues. I agreed with him. I knew they were. I had studied quite a bit and understood the anatomy of the throat.

Since 1975, I'd had thyroid issues that had gone undiagnosed for more than 20 years. In 1996 I was placed on thyroid medication when my thyroid score was at 18+. I thought I understood thyroid issues, but I would come to look at thyroid illness in a different way as my research continued. It was all tied together. I just wasn't aware of it until much later.

I went home with mixed feelings. While I was grateful that the new ENT doctor had visually verified the severity of the throat damage, I was also starting to come out of my sad resignation of being ashamed for being so sick.

By the time I arrived home I was livid. I was angry about being made to feel so ashamed for being ill. I was angry that doctors became hostile when I stated the facts as I remembered them. I was angry at not being believed. And I was devastated that my doctors were so indifferent to my suffering.

I couldn't figure out why my medical records didn't reflect what the doctors told me verbally. It would be some time before I found out that what is told to a patient is not necessarily what is written in the chart. Medical charts are written with as little as possible in them. What I did not know was that no ENT ever wrote the words "laryngopharyngeal reflux disease" even though the term was used several times to me in their offices.

When I got home, I cried from anger and frustration. I cried from the loneliness of an illness for which there are no answers and from the fact that even the doctors shun you. I realized that the way the new GI had treated me was abuse of a patient. I wrote an email to the ENT who had just observed my seared throat. "I am writing to inform you that I am requesting that you facilitate a new GI specialist for me IMMEDIATELY! Please find me a GI that believes the patient. If this is not done I will report what has happened to me to the Chief of Staff."

I was answered immediately and a new GI was provided, but I knew after much research that very little is known about laryngopharyngeal reflux (LPR), even though it is a very common illness. It is difficult to diagnose and equally difficult to treat. And I knew that I had a very severe case of LPR. The University of California, Davis has an excellent online article on LPR, but it merely describes the symptoms and how the throat looks. It does not discuss the root cause of the illness because I don't think doctors really know what causes it.

My next few appointments were with radiology and an endocrinology specialist for the thyroid growth and a new GI for my burning ulcerated throat. The Endocrinologist did many tests and thoroughly reviewed my entire chart. He was at a loss as to why I had a searing throat, but said indeed my thyroid needed to be removed immediately.

The newest GI that replaced the last one was young and pleasant. I noticed that she wasn't typing on the computer keyboard like the other doctors. She sat in the middle of the examination room and actually looked at me. She said quietly, "We are sorry. We believe you now."

I was angry, but I didn't show it. It wasn't her fault. The new GI was so young. I decided that maybe she would think outside the box and help me research. I was in the dark and taking stabs at research, but after months of reading about a particular area, I always concluded that it didn't fit my particular set of anatomical problems. My issues centered on the upper esophageal sphincter (UES) and there is no surgery to correct a malfunctioning UES.

But I have to say I learned a great deal and became a bit of a "home scholar" on my condition.

In the next two months, the new GI gave me several medications to try. Each one left me with exponentially unrelenting throat pain. It was hopeless.

I brought my GI about six articles on laryngopharyngeal reflux, downloaded from one of the nearby University of California teaching hospitals. She seemed surprised to see them. I also brought her the first GI's diagnosis, written by hand on her imprinted name medical pad: *laryngopharyngeal reflux*. The new GI specialist stared at the diagnosis, but made no comment. I asked her to place it in my medical file. She said she would. She asked me where I got the articles on LPR. I told her they were on the internet from the nearby University of California site. I had simply downloaded and printed them from the website of the nearby teaching hospital. She seemed surprised. She told me that she had interned at UC Davis and had never heard of that term. She asked me whether she could keep the articles. I told her I brought the articles for her.

On several other visits, my GI told me that some doctors didn't believe in the laryngopharyngeal reflux diagnosis. I was surprised, very surprised. It is a common illness that is often misdiagnosed as allergies or asthma for many patients over many years. Some patient go for decades with an allergy or asthma diagnosis when in fact it is a Laryngopharyngeal Reflux they have. At least, that is what the latest research indicates. I told the newest GI that the LPR merely describes the symptoms, not the cause, and that my medical presentation fit every symptom of LPR. I was 100% sure I had LPR, but I couldn't figure out how to get better.

At this point, I asked the GI if she would help me obtain a referral to the local teaching hospital to see whether a second opinion could be obtained. She said she would relay the request to her department head.

I waited and waited for months. I continued all my appointments between the specialties: ENT, GI and Endocrinology with the young GI doctor leading, month after month, waiting for an answer.

As Christmas 2010 approached, I kept myself together by swallowing anything and everything over the counter to neutralize acid and sooth my seared throat. Nothing helped. Not even strong pain medication. I stopped pain medication when I realized I was still in wrenching pain and had developed severe constipation. I reasoned that I seared with or without medication so I probably should not burden my body with medicines that did nothing to help me, but it was hard. It was minute by minute endurance challenge to get through each minute, hour and day. Nights were so long. The pain was so difficult my sleep was reduced to one minute at a time. I don't know how I managed to not fall apart. The condition was getting worse and I began to feel acid burning in my back and the front of my chest. I would shake from pain and have to walk through the house. There was no sitting down or resting. Nothing helped me escape the ravages of a severe case of LPR.

CHAPTER 9

JANUARY 2011 THROUGH JULY 2011

Things still looked pretty hopeless for my situation and condition. I still had not scheduled a biopsy on my throat nor had my thyroid removal. I knew I would have to do so soon. I just couldn't bring myself to go into surgery because of the pain I was in and I knew the medications for surgery would make my searing more than I could bear at this point. So I delayed as much as I could as I searched for something to give me relief.

I had been losing one to two pounds daily for the last month and I knew I was on a path to a slow painful death. In fact, I calculated at my rate of losing of weight that by 80 pounds I would probably die from starvation. I knew I had to figure out what was wrong with me quickly. I told my doctors about my loss of weight, but they were silent and at a loss as to what to do for me. My sister called me one day and gently told me I had to prepare things in case I died from this illness. It was hard to hear, but I told her I had already divided up my jewelry for my daughters and put their names on the envelopes. It was one of the toughest things to face, knowing that one cannot stop an illness. I was resigned, but just stubborn enough not to want to accept eventually dying from this mysterious illness that no one knew how to treat.

One day in January 2011, my neighbor Kathy came to visit, bringing a newly purchased box of probiotics, which she said might help me. I took several capsules that first day and for the first time, I had a slight relief. Reading about probiotics, I learned that a large quantity could be taken without harm, so I felt I had nothing to lose. I swallowed more and more and felt a small improvement of about five percent. I still burned terribly because my throat was so raw with ulcer acid burns. The acid vapor never stopped floating up to my throat 24 hours a day. My raw scorched throat just never got a chance to heal. It was non-stop hydrochloric acid vapor on my throat 24/7. I have never been so scared in my life.

I told my new young GI that probiotics had given me a tiny bit of relief. She seemed surprised, but said that she could prescribe medical-strength probiotics for me, capsules containing 900 billion active cells each. She said I could take up to four packets a day. I did and experienced more improvement – maybe 15 percent. I was surprised, and so was she.

At my next ENT appointment, however, my throat still looked the same. That was hard to hear. Under pressure from the ENT, I reluctantly agreed to the throat biopsy and the removal of my thyroid. Both were scheduled for February 2011. It was all I could do to pull my shaking body together and go in for the surgery.

The biopsy results on both the throat and removal of the thyroid came back negative. It was such good news. So far, I did not have cancer of the throat or thyroid, but that good news was tempered by the searing throat pain that remained constantly with me. Dealing with the pain was exhausting. I often felt that if I didn't wake up from the fitful sleep that gave me a moment of reprieve, it would be okay. But I had so much to live for. I stubbornly continued to use the World Wide Web to seek answers. The negative biopsy results meant that I had more time to keep researching and piecing together the root cause of my illness, if one could be found.

During this time I stumbled across message boards that I became so grateful for. I had been reading LPR message boards online, reading accounts by people from all around the world with similar cases like mine. Some had suffered severely for a decade and longer. I was surprised to read that so many of them had also been accused by their doctors of causing their condition. Many of them said their doctors had become upset with them. Many said family members had turned on them, blaming them. One woman with severe LPR said she was losing hope. In one message board entry, she said her husband had planned a beautiful anniversary dinner, and she wept uncontrollable at the restaurant. He was so happy to surprise her, but she couldn't eat because of her throat pain.

I read of mothers searching for help. Their babies and toddlers had LPR and they were getting nowhere with the doctors. Their children were suffering.

One man in his twenties with LPR for five years said his doctors couldn't help him and his family thought he had mental health issues. He was unable to work or go to college and his life was falling apart. I cried when I read those accounts. All of us LPR patients seemed to be in a hopeless situation. We got blamed for a very real and debilitating illness.

I could identify with many of the people on the message boards. They encouraged me and kept me from the darkness of knowing that I only had a small window of time to figure this out.

It was incredibly sad.

But the message boards did help me a great deal. I realized I was quite sane and not doing this to myself. There had to be a concrete reason for this to happen, but what was it?

I read about babies and children had LPR, as well as young adults who were losing their speaking voice, even professional singers who could no longer sing. One women in a Scandinavian country wrote that her husband died from LPR because he couldn't eat or swallow water. He eventually withered away and died in horrible pain. That terrified me. My research became even more urgent. I knew that I was in a serious health situation and that time was of the essence.

Each day I read these entries I began to see a pattern. And it occurred to me that there had to be one common denominator for LPR – something that all these different people around the world, young and old, had in common.

The research on LPR/GERD seemed to indicate that LPR is similar to GERD, which occurs when the lower esophageal sphincter (LES) – the valve between the esophagus and the stomach – allows stomach contents into the esophagus. But I was beginning to question the theory that this was caused by food and drink as I continued my research. The message board's participants' ages were all over the place. How can a baby or child or even young adult have time to wear out their sphincters in the esophagus? That was my nagging question. What was the common denominator for all of us? It seemed obvious to me there had to be one root cause to this. I kept reading and slowly building layers of knowledge. Though I had no science or medical background, I was an administrator in my career with a Public Administration Masters degree. I am by no means someone who would be expected to figure out something no doctor could figure out. That was also part of the desperation as I studied. I could have been wasting my time, but I was compelled to learn as much as I could until the day I died from this horrible illness.

I was aware that all the literature on GERD/LPR advising not to eat certain foods as it may cause reflux. I could understand the logic of avoiding tomatoes, raw onions, raw garlic and hot spices, but why was my throat burning on plain water and very low-acid bland food? I not only followed the recommendations on what not to eat, but I ate so little, and I had the Nissen fundoplication that should have fixed the problem. After all, I had a new PH score of 0.40! Nearly a perfect PH study.

It would be a while before I could connect the dots and solve the mystery, but I held on to the observation that people of all ages got LPR. So there had to be one factor that was common to all, I reasoned. I became a detective on the LPR mystery.

As the months went by, the probiotics gave me some very small consistent relief. My GI doctor thought that it changed the pH of my stomach acid. I think she was correct.

And she told me after a pH study that showed my score had gone from 40 to 0.4 that she thought the surgery had helped me, even if I felt worse. But why did I feel 100x worse after the surgery? It was a huge mystery to me and was literally driving me crazy thinking about it.

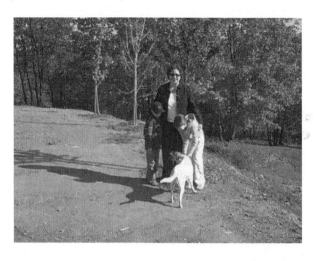

Figure 3 Author with her grandchildren and dog, Bella Mia, hiding her debilitating illness.

In the spring of 2011, I decided that if I was going to die early, I was going to go out doing the things I loved. And the joy of a lifetime for me was watching my grandchildren swimming in the new pool. I pushed myself to do the normal things of life with my family. I also decided to join three groups and although it was hard sitting still in meetings because I usually paced the floor to walk off my pain, the meetings gave me a feeling of purpose other than just dealing with pain.

And then in early May 2011, I developed two other physical ailments. One was severe shoulder-joint pain on both sides. I could not raise my arms an inch without excruciating pain. That meant I had to wash my hair, dress myself, do my housework and shop without lifting my arms. I tried to hide this from everyone. I was now more ashamed than ever, thinking I was literally falling apart and that it was my fault according to the doctor's implications earlier. I also developed incontinence that got worse as the days passed. I was quietly panicking, but there was no one to turn to.

At the same time, I began to burn worse in the center of my back downward. I was sure that the acid was now eating through the tissue of the thick lower part of my esophagus. My fear intensified and I felt hopeless as I deteriorated.

My last, faint hope was the possibility of getting a second opinion on the LPR from the teaching hospital, so I kept asking my GI for any news on my request.

CHAPTER 10

AUGUST 2011

In August 2011, after waiting for seven months for an answer about the second-opinion referral, I called my GI again. She said I could see the head GI at a hospital about two-and-a-half hours away. Would I be willing to go? I said yes enthusiastically as by now I would have done anything to get better. It was a hard trip as I was in so much pain and every moment in route to the hospital was hard.

At the hospital, 45 minutes late, this new young GI entered my exam room. He seemed totally indifferent. Basically all he did was shrug his shoulders at every question I asked. He told me I had to learn to live with my throat condition. He said he didn't know what I had, but it wasn't LPR. I said, "Doctor, LPR was the diagnosis I was given in the San Francisco Bay Area, and I had a surgery based on it. All the literature states exactly my symptoms and it all points to LPR." I then asked what he thought I had, if it was not LPR? He shrugged his shoulders and said he didn't know.

All I could think was that the medical professionals just didn't want to spend any more money on me. My illness was untreatable. I asked the GI if he would please give me a referral to a local teaching hospital. He said that it wasn't his call. He stated that it was my local GI's call. I didn't believe that.

My recent research had led me to wonder about my vagus nerve, which supplies nerve fibers to the throat and digestive system. I asked the GI whether he thought I had a problem with the vagus nerve. That question apparently angered him. "OF COURSE YOU DO!" It was a strange moment for me. I had come to the private conclusion that the vagus nerve was not the cause of my throat/head pain, but I wanted to understand everything about my condition. I needed his opinion, but my questions were making him agitated.

Trying to ignore his shrugging shoulders and keep my dignity as I was graveling for someone to care about me, I asked whether he had ever seen a case like mine (he nodded he had), and whether any new treatments were on the horizon. He shrugged his shoulders again indifferently. "No, it will be ten years before they have an answer for what you have. You have to learn to live with it."

At that point I could see he was sick and tired of me. I thanked him and pretended I didn't see his disdain for my taking up his time. I acknowledged to the doctor that I knew he was a very busy person. I was trying so hard to keep some dignity in the discussion. I asked him if he would keep me in mind should he hear of any new therapies that could be tried. He said okay, but his reply was hollow. On my ride home, I wondered how many patients go through this kind of treatment when they have a chronic condition and how many are blamed for their illness.

Later, I was told by my local GI that the man I had just seen had denied me a second opinion outside of my provider. She restated that the doctors didn't know what I had. She would not be following me any longer, as there was nothing more she could do for me. There are no words to describe how that feels.

CHAPTER 11

AUGUST 2011

When I got home, I sat at my computer, wondering how long it might be before damage to the tissues and nerves of my throat led to bleeding or even cancer. I knew my condition of acid hitting the throat had caused ulcer burns and I had been like this for 2 ½ years. The acid vapor was slowly wearing away at my throat nerves that went up into the head and down throughout the body. I knew from my personal research that if one deteriorates further, it can be quite a serious situation.

Then something about my ongoing research began circulating in my mind. My problem seemed centered on esophageal sphincters, in particular the Upper Esophageal Sphincter (UES), a muscular tube at the top of the esophagus, connecting the pharynx. The lower sphincter had been tightened by the surgery, but there was no surgery for the upper one. Or at least I couldn't find any in my internet searches. And I had studied the anatomy of the esophagus and was able, as a non-scientist, to surmise that there was a normal acid vapor puff, that we all have, that usually doesn't get past the Upper Esophageal Sphincter (LES). I was beginning to think that my problem centered on the Upper Esophageal Sphincter (UES) not closing off that small bit of acid vapor puff that is natural part of digestion in all of us.

I was formulating a theory that my upper sphincter had an atrophy of sorts. They had fixed the Lower Esophageal Sphincter (LES) with the Nissen fundoplication surgery, but the Upper Esophageal Sphincter (UES) had no surgery that could be done to tighten it. I thought about that common theory I had on all ages getting LPR. What was the common denominator?

All this time I had been doing research using the word "sphincters". Realizing in that moment, sitting at my computer about to do more research, that sphincters was just another word for small muscles, I entered in my computer a query that would not only change the course of my illness, but would shed light on many of the other illnesses we suffer from in modern society. I entered in the World Wide Web: "*What strengthens muscles?*" It was that simple.

The answers opened up a world of science for me. There were many articles that popped up on the web referencing muscles but there was one that caught my eye. It said athletes use Vitamin D to strengthen muscles and that vitamin D was actually a hormone made from the sun. I blinked when I saw the word "hormone". I had some experience with the incredible impact of a hormone on health, the thyroid hormone. My heart raced. What if this could help strengthen my upper esophageal sphincter (UES)? Even if it helped a small bit, it was worth the try.

And then I stopped and thought, "Where had I been for six decades? How is it that I didn't know that vitamin D is made by the sun on one's skin?"

It suddenly hit me like a bolt of lightning, a lot of people call it the Ah Ha moment, that I had avoided the sun since I was in my early twenties because I had read over and over that the sun was harmful. Could there be a connection between this and the severity of my illness? I was dumbstruck. I had believed all the warnings in the media since the early 1970s about how harmful the sun was!

As a result, I realized, my body might have permanent damage because of lack of sunshine.

And then it occurred to me that just before I had the fundoplication surgery in May 2009, I had stopped taking calcium citrate. I ran to find the bottle in my cabinet. I still had it. It had a little Vitamin D in it, 600 international units. Could that be why I got worse after the surgery? That 600 IU of D a day was all that I was getting just before surgery. From the moment that I stopped calcium citrate/vitamin D pill I realized I was not getting any Vitamin D, either from the sun or the citrate pill and that is why I got worse from LPR after surgery. Together with knowing that I shied away from the sun for 40 years made me think that I might have found an answer.

Connecting the dots further, I thought about the bone pain I had suffered for 20 years that only stopped when I took calcium citrate. Now I realized it was not the calcium citrate that stopped the bone pain, it was that small bit, 600 IU, of Vitamin D in the calcium capsules that had stopped the pain. When I stopped taking the calcium citrate and D before the fundoplication surgery, I was probably already on an empty tank of vitamin D. It now made sense why I got worse after stopping the calcium/vitamin D vitamin. It explained why I got worse after surgery-I was not getting any D at all.

As I researched, everything fell into place. Apparently all the illnesses of my life are directly linked to low D levels or at least that is my personal theory.

I continued to read all I could find about vitamin D to figure out how to treat myself. I had lost all faith and trust in my doctors. I still feel they work hard and are well educated, but I also realize that diagnoses are often educated guesses and that drug-based medicine and surgery may not always be what is needed.

None of my doctors really looked for the cause of my illnesses. If drugs and surgery didn't work, I was on my own. To my knowledge, no doctor had ever tested me for vitamin D deficiency. What a travesty!

The "common thread theory" that I had for my illness that tied babies, young people, adults and seniors together was coming into focus. I felt sure that vitamin D had to be the common denominator I had been looking for.

My thoughts floated back to 1996, when I was 44 years old and sleeping a lot. In fact, over a three-month period I was setting an alarm clock after breakfast on the weekends so that I could go back to sleep. I had to push myself out of bed at noon and again at six p.m. My husband urged me to see a doctor. When I did, the doctor discovered I was suffering from Hashimoto's disease – a condition in which the immune system attacks the thyroid – and prescribed a thyroid hormone.

When I took the thyroid hormone for the first time, my arms and whole body felt as though I had a huge rubber band stretched across me. I suspect that this indicated that I was quite in need of thyroid hormone. A year later, when I had my eyes tested for glasses, the doctor exclaimed, "What have you been doing since I last saw you? Your eyes have improved considerably!" At first I could not think of anything that was different. Then I remembered the thyroid hormone I was given a year before. "Oh! That is why your eyes have improved so much," the vision doctor said.

From my experience with that thyroid hormone, I knew that D hormone would have a profound impact on my LPR. I felt it in my bones – no pun intended. Much later I drilled down into Vitamin D research and realized that thyroid illness is an autoimmune illness and directly linked back to low D for too many years.

In my research on vitamin D, I learned that I should take a lab test to determine the levels of D in my system. I also read that B12 deficiency can cause serious medical issues and goes hand in hand with low D scores. I emailed my primary doctor within minutes of putting all this together, and without telling her why (I was beyond explaining or asking permission for anything), asked her to have two lab tests waiting for me in the morning: D and B12.

I then ordered from a reputable online company several levels of international units of D3. The literature indicated that there were two types of D: D2 and D3. It seemed from the literature that D3 was the better of the two.

When the vitamin D arrived a few days later, I had already carefully decided how much D3 to take, based on my research: the formula was 35 IU of D3 times each pound of body weight. To be safe, I subtracted 2,000 IU from that sum. I was worried about taking too much D3. I had read many articles by doctors, warning against the dangers of too much D. It would take another two years of researching before I decided to add that 2,000 IU back. I now firmly believe that there is too much worry on D3. Based on the literature, anything 10,000 IU or below for an adult is very safe. Now I base the dosage on how I feel and on my lab tests and my weight. As time went on, it occurred to me when I read the scare articles on vitamin D that no doctor **ever** seemed too worried about the dangers of extremely high doses of proton pump inhibitors (PPIs) and dangerous pain medications or surgery. How ironic.

After only one day of supplementing with D3, I was stunned the next morning to find that my locked up shoulder blades and the incontinence disappeared. The burning in my back disappeared very slowly and steadily over the next two years (I believe in addition to LPR I was developing GERD with the burning pain in my back). This was a stunning outcome. Over the next two years, the LPR pain lifted slowly and faded away to an improvement of close to 100 percent. The locked up shoulder blades and incontinence disappeared over night, never to return. Simply stunning!

Today I still am amazed that, after all my consultations with doctors, I ended up diagnosing and treating myself. I am just a patient with no medical or science background. How is it possible that my highly educated doctors missed this? How is it that the endocrinologist I was seeing didn't test my D levels? In fact, why isn't D testing part of routine preventive medicine? An endocrinologist's specialty is hormones of the body! I wondered how many other people this happens to and I thought about all the years that this was missed on me. I think about how it is missed on all of us. There are no words when I think about the unnecessary suffering for something so simple to fix.

The laboratory test confirmed what I had suspected – I was suffering from vitamin D deficiency. My first D score was a US lab score of 25 ng/mL. According to the Vitamin

D scientists, a score between zero and 30 indicates deficiency; 31 to 39 is insufficient; 40 to 80 is sufficient; and anything above 150 is toxic. My research indicates that anything under 40 US ng/mL suggests a risk of developing a serious illness. I still shudder when I look at a D deficiency/illness chart. (The US uses different lab scoring than the UK/Canada. Very important to know when reading articles.)

I think of all the people of the planet walking around with low D levels, and I know they are in jeopardy – walking time bombs for any illness. How many children and young adults have had their lives ruined by an illness that is preventable? It is unconscionable.

In the spring of 2012, US lab D charts dropped the "low-normal" score to 20 (from 30)! I was incredulous! That means that some doctors will tell patients with a score of 21 that they "fall within normal limits." To my limited understanding this is a travesty. It is not normal. At the very minimum, people should be aiming for a score of 40-60 US ng/mL.

The big question about my own score was: why wasn't my D score lower than 25? My first twenty years was spent growing up in San Francisco and it was shrouded in fog a great deal of the time. In fact I had spent most of my life at the 37th latitude on the planet, which increases the odds of low D score. In addition to that already huge risk factor, I had avoided the sun for 40 years as an adult and had worked inside an office. And then I thought back to the spring of 2011. By being outside in the sunshine with my grandchildren around the new pool from April to August 2011 (I had thrown my caution about sunshine on my skin out as I wanted to enjoy my last few months with my grandchildren). Those five months, from April to August in 2011 in the sunshine probably brought my D score up to 25 by the end of summer. I suspect I spent most of my life hovering at a US D score of 15 ng/mL.

Next I had to understand why the incontinence disappeared within 24 hours of starting D3. I learned that the bladder has a sphincter that opens and closes, allowing urine to flow or stop. It hit me that all our organs have sphincters – even our intestines are one big muscle. And vitamin (hormone) D strengthens all muscles and cells of the body, whether in the veins, arteries, gut, esophagus, legs, face or heart. All muscles and cells need D. And so do bones, cartilage and tendons.

I learned that being overweight causes even lower D levels as the fat cells take up the D and store it, leaving the body running on an empty D tank. I read that D moves calcium from the gut to where it belongs in the body. That the esophagus is completely lined in D receptors. That the esophagus cells are very similar to cartilage and bone cells. That bone regeneration needs D. That all our cells are "held" together by Vitamin D. That without high enough levels of D, cells develop gaps and start to fall apart.

I learned that D strengthens muscle tone. That "muscle twitch" diminishes without high enough D levels. That probably explains why I had weak legs since I was in my early 40s. And why my Upper Esophageal Sphincter (UES) was not closing off the normal stomach vapor as it was intended to do. It had lost "muscle twitch". Together with the esophagus not receiving enough D, the end result was my esophagus that was not functioning properly due to low D levels for too many decades. Probably since utero. An unnerving realization. I could assume I had permanent damage from a lifetime of low weak sunshine at the 37+ latitude on the planet and low D scores throughout a lifetime.

I couldn't help asking myself why isn't there laboratory testing for D levels front and center in preventive medicine? And why aren't evolutionary needs tests inexpensive (or free) so that everyone can get one? I have formulated some private opinions, but it is hard to say them out loud because I'm not a doctor and don't have the credentials to talk about this professionally. I can only relay to my readers my personal story and theories about my illnesses and recovery, even though I'm not cured. I am certainly in a "remission" of sorts, as long as I keep my D score hovering at US score of 80 ng/mL.

As for my LPR, I noticed an immediate lifting of the throat pain when I took Vitamin D. It was not an immediate recovery, but it did get better after two years on D3. With each week that passed, I felt better and better. By then I had stopped seeing all my specialists. I had spent money on the visits, had taken expensive medications and had undergone a major surgery – only to get worse and meet nothing but silence and indifference and the implication that it was stress causing my illness. And that I could do something about it. Yes, I was so angry to know that I suffered for something, which was so simple to fix. But I am grateful to have discovered it before I lost my life. I often think if people only knew, they would run, not walk, to get tested and they would educate themselves on the science of D and sunshine. It is a matter of life and death….literally.

After three months on vitamin (hormone) D, I decided to go for another scope to find out how my throat looked. I noticed that over the previous three months the pain had gone away in my neck and back of my head, although I still had throat discomfort.

The ENT greeted me with his usual pleasant and friendly manner. "You look different!" he told me. I knew I did because the LPR pain was fading. When you are in pain for months on end, your whole face changes. As the ENT doctor scoped the upper part of my throat, he said, "Your upper throat is still angry but slightly better." I was so happy to hear that. I had read multiple ulcer burns in the throat take a long time to heal. I said, "Yes, it still feels rough and hurts, but it's better."

Then the ENT went deeper into my throat and looked at the back of my throat where he had done the biopsy in February 2011. "Gosh, what have you been doing?" he asked. "The spot I biopsied is completely healed!" I quietly said, "I'm taking vitamin D3." From that moment on, the ENT did not make another comment. On my next visit, he told me my throat was better, but made no other comments and did not ask any questions about my remarkable recovery. I never quite understood that and probably never will. And I noticed that his office now contained LPR pamphlets. I was quite surprised as they had told me they didn't believe in the diagnosis of LPR, which is difficult to comprehend because a diagnosis of LPR doesn't imply what causes it. It merely describes the symptoms.

The other improvements in my health and appearance are worth noting here. The dark rings under my eyes that I had to use cover-up makeup on had now disappeared. My skin looked better. The varicose veins in my legs that I had thought might eventually need surgery completely disappeared. Much to my surprise, my sleep improved immensely. The muscles of my legs got stronger. I used to struggle to climb stairs (even at 40 years old); now at 65 years old, I do so with no problem (and I'm 65 at the moment). My wrists use to be swollen. They have lost the puffiness. It is all remarkable. I still can't quite get over how lucky I was to stumble across that muscle/athlete article on vitamin D.

It would be some time before I discovered the Vitamin D scientists of the world. My favorite science writer on this subject is Dr. Oliver Gillie of the UK. His articles and clarity opened a new world of understanding as to what happened to me. The Grassroots Health Organization of California is full of the newest research on the subject that is another wonderful resource. And of course Vitamin D Wiki shows all the known illnesses related to low D. If you notice, my illness of Laryngopharyngeal Reflux (LPR) is not listed, so I suspect there is so much that is unknown about illness and its relationship to low D scores. And there is nothing listed on leaking bladder or locked up shoulder blades, but those illnesses disappeared overnight, never to return, on one dosing of D3!

The science of D has existed on the books for many decades. In the 1930's children had rickets and cod liver oil was used and the doctors also noticed that not only did ricket cases reduce substantially, but diabetes in children declined when the cod liver oil was used.

The practice of testing for D and keeping D scores high enough is not part of routine preventive care. It should be. As a global population we have moved from the forests and having our skin exposed to the sun to indoor dwellings and clothing covering our skin and now we spend more time in front of computers and television screens. Fewer of us work outside. Many of us are afraid of the sun because of scare stories about cancer. And many people lather on the sunscreen. We might be modern humans, but we have never lost the biological need for sunshine. Evolutionary needs of the human body should be front and center in a doctor's medical training. There is no doubt in my mind that every single one of us are at great risk not having high enough D scores. We should be checked as part of preventive medicine from utero until old age. The travesty of this lack of process in medicine today must be something every patient demands in their health care examinations. Especially women and men who plan to start a family. A child deserves the best chance for a long life with minimal illnesses throughout their lifetime.

CHAPTER 12

2012...2013...2014...2015...2016...2017

It has now been about six and half years since I started sunning and keeping my D scores hovering at 80 ng/ml (US scoring). D scientists recommend aiming for a D score range of 40-60 US ng/mL. Because I believe I have severe atrophy of all the muscles of my body, and that the sphincters of my throat are severely affected by lack of high enough D scores throughout my lifetime, I need to keep my D score higher than most. I have permanent damage to my muscle tone due to a lifetime of low D. When my D score falls to 62 US ng/mL score the LPR returns slowly. There are not many times in life that a patient happens across something so profound that it changes one's entire quality of life and perspective.

In my case, discovering vitamin (hormone) D3 and sunning in the nude has had a positive effect on turning around a devastating illness doctors were unable to diagnose or help me with. It improved the quality of my health and how I think about the human body and its evolutionary needs.

One of the things that struck me as I have researched the last six or so years is that for decades the general population was not informed about the importance of vitamin D and sunshine – they were told for decades to avoid the sun. And they are still told to wear skin protection. If one thinks about that, it really is totally against our evolutionary needs. There are vitamin D scientists who think that the number of all types of illness would drop significantly if everyone kept their D levels closer to a score of 40-60 ng/mL.

I now live at 38 latitude so I am acutely aware that the sun does not produce D on the skin from mid-September through mid-April at my latitude. I also know that I am older and my skin does not produce D like when I was 19 years old. I try to schedule vacations every two months in the winter from mid-September through mid-April below the 30th latitude on the planet.

When I look back, there is one regret I have. I should have started taking D3 at higher loading doses. Yet even at such a low loading dose, I still got better from two illnesses within 24 hours: the leaking bladder and the locked up shoulder blades. The Laryngopharyngeal Reflux (LPR) took longer to fade away because my dosing of D3 was too low. There is not a day that goes by that I don't think of all the people who are suffering and are sick or have died for lack of this very inexpensive and easy-to-treat evolutionary need. And my heart is broken for them. Who am I, I ask myself, to speak on this subject? How can I help? And that is how I have come to tell you my story of illness, discovery and recovery.

The literature on Vitamin D indicates that it is best to get it directly from the sun during the high sun in the afternoon. For those of us in daylight savings time that is 1 p.m. after spring. However, most of us live at latitudes where the sun's rays are too weak part of the year to produce vitamin D on our skin; therefore, supplements are needed to avoid risk of a wide range of illnesses.

One way of figuring out the correct dosage is this formula: 1,000 IU of D3 for each 25 pounds of weight. In other words, a person weighing 125 pounds may need up to 5,000 IU of D3 a day. And if their D tank is on empty they may need more for a little while to get their D score to at least 50. It is important to test often until you get a sense of what keeps you at a decent D score.

I do a lab test twice a year because it is essential that I keep my D score high enough to keep my illnesses in "remission". I aim for taking a D test twice a year, once at the end of February (end of winter) and once at the end of September (end of summer). I do it through my health-care provider or Grassroots Health or any certified lab in your community can do it as well. It does cost for the test, but as patients, let us work toward advocating to make basic D testing fully covered by our health-care insurance. It is so important that world health care experts to push for health education and prevention protocols that will allow everyone to obtain D testing free. D awareness needs to become part of preventive medicine.

Ideally D3 should be offered free to citizens everywhere. I often contemplate how much money could be saved worldwide if we could cut illnesses down drastically? And how much suffering could be eliminated? Think about governments saving trillions of dollars a year. What citizens and governments could do with funds like that to improve the quality of life! People would actually be able to have something saved and invested for old age. Our government could do things that helped people improve their lives and their communities. Education could be free worldwide. I sincerely believe that if testing and education on obtaining high enough D levels were part of our preventive health-care system, it would change almost every person's life on the planet.

The weight of bad health, due to modern living behaviors, will disrupt nations' budgets and cause economic upheaval. The common person is spending too much for health care as well as suffering with marginal health. And much of that suffering is preventable. My opinion from the aggregate of research I've done is that all illnesses could be reduced by 50-75% if we had adequate D scores.

Populations in the sweet zone of the equator are now more and more inclined to have low levels of vitamin D. They are acquiring the modern behavior of staying inside all day long and wearing clothes that cover the body. My grandmother was born and lived in Managua, Nicaragua below the 31st latitude. She died of a stroke at the age of 55. I never got to meet her.

I had been wondering why people living near the equator have been found to have low levels of vitamin D since they lived at the sweet zone of excellent UVB light on their skin and I couldn't help thinking about my Grandmother Elena who lived in Managua, Nicaragua from 1900-1955. I asked my mother about my Grandmother Elena's sun exposure. My mother thought a bit and said Grandmother Elena had not spent any time outdoors. My mother said, "She never went in the sun. She stayed inside all the time running her shoe business from morning into the late night trying to make enough money to feed eight children."

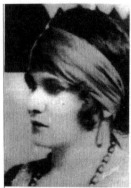

Figure 4 Author's maternal Grandmother Elena (1900-1955). Managua, Nicaragua

Grandmother Elena died from a stroke. Could it have been low D? The loss to her eight children was immeasurable, and I never got to meet her.

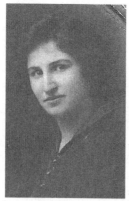

*Figure 5 Author's paternal Grandmother Eva (1896-1934).
International Falls, Minnesota.*

Grandmother Eva lost two babies in utero, back to back, which caused a cascade of medical attempts to save her life. Could her loss of babies been caused by low D levels? She lived at a high latitude on the planet for D creation on her skin. Her loss was devastating for her husband and four young children, and I never got to meet her.

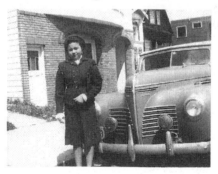

*Figure 6 Author's mother Demis in 1947 (1930-...).
San Francisco Bay Area.*

Demis developed rheumatoid arthritis. Could it be due low D?

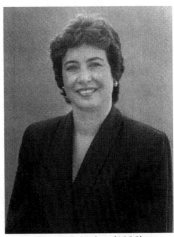

Figure 7 Author (1996)

Could a lifetime of low D levels have caused me a lifetime of progressive illness; such as, anemia, bad memory, menorrhagia, amenorrhea, tonsillectomy, two C-sections, bone pain, weak muscles, thyroid illness and removal, melanoma, osteomalacia, high blood pressure, severe sleep apnea, two 1 year periods of severe plantar fasciitis, arthritis of the knees, laryngopharyngeal reflux, locked up shoulder blades and incontinence? The literature indicates it is a real possibility based on what science knows today.

The literature indicates that D is made on the skin when the sun hits it directly. The sun is the first and best way to obtain higher D levels. But when one lives above the 31st latitude, especially during months when the sun's rays are weak, supplementing with D3 may be necessary. I know taking a pill is not the same as the sun rays on my skin, but from my firsthand experience with laryngopharyngeal reflux, locked up shoulder joints, incontinence and burning GERD in my back being reversed, I will settle for D3 capsules when I have no other options.

Vitamin D scientists are studying how much D to take and they are struggling to get the Institute of Medicine (IOM) (an American non-profit organization that gives advice on national health and medical issues) to change current guidelines on optimal D levels. I have gleaned from the literature that some D scientists believe that if you have been sick, it might not hurt to get a D score to the 70-80 range. I notice that when my D score starts to fall to 62, the LPR starts to slowly come back. I try to keep my level closer to 80 ng/ml. It is where I feel the best.

The literature indicates that when one reaches the age of 50, the body makes 70 percent less D on the skin than on a 19- year-old. In other words, age substantially reduces our ability to synthesize D on our skin. So that is an important issue to weigh as one considers D levels and supplementing.

Another variable is the color of one's skin. Because I'm lighter skinned, I take a timer with me and sun 15-20 minutes on each side of my body. Those with darker skin can stay in the sun longer so that the sun's rays can penetrate the skin. It is why darker skin people have higher rates of cancer, heart disease and metabolic illnesses. Their D levels are chronically low decade after decade.

From an evolutionary perspective, darker skinned people are in a latitude that is different than their skin tones and therefore they are at greater risk for more chronic debilitating illnesses of all types.

I am so heartbroken for all the lost lives and suffering of people with something so simple and inexpensive to treat. Maybe it's because I felt so doomed knowing I would eventually die from all my health issues and no one could help me. I felt utterly hopeless to stop the cascading illnesses that were piling up and I was ashamed because I was made to feel that I was causing it to myself with "stress" even though I had none.

In December 2014, I read that President Obama had reflux of the throat. I remember thinking he is probably low on D. I read a few weeks later he was in Hawaii and golfing. I was so happy to read that he was in the stronger sunshine of Hawaii. I believe sunshine below the 31st latitude is the best thing for helping with the unbearable pain of acid vapor in the throat and the slow progression of all illnesses that pile up when D scores are low.

I suspect the singer Prince (who I just loved his music!) may have had LPR and was put on medications, which may have cascaded to his untimely death. I couldn't help thinking that it may have been related to low D scores too. It is my theory but a haunting one. I remember reading in an article that Prince's chef said that he was having problem with reflux and eating, and if he experienced anything like my case, it cascades into more and more medications. It is a slow painful spiral down. I read that Prince lived at a high latitude, which further makes me think there could be a link to low D score, but like I said, it is just my theory.

I did write President Obama and First Lady Michelle Obama in 2016 to warn them and ask to have the issue studied. People with darker skin are at greater risk as darker skin is a natural sunscreen. It doesn't help people with darker skin tone to live at the higher weaker D latitude zones for making D on the skin.

I read that wearing clothes was one of the biggest problems in getting enough D produced on our skin. The back is where most of the D is made. So I did something previously unthinkable: I sun in the nude. I'm lucky, I have a patio that is private. Not everyone around the world has a small space of privacy. We need to make our rooftops places to sun in privacy. At least we need to be aware that removing enough clothes while we get safe sunshine is critical to quality health and length of life

I've come to the conclusion after years of studying D science that I may have permanent damage from too many decades without direct sun on my skin. Because of the latitude where I was brought up, I suspect I even had low D since childhood – maybe even since my mother became pregnant with me. The childhood anemia that carried into my adulthood is an autoimmune illness that may be caused by low D levels.

During the last forty years, I have been suffering with weak muscles. In my early forties my knees and legs ached, and sometimes my legs and knees felt wobbly and unstable. Each time I told my doctors about this, they would give me a sheet of paper with exercises that they said would strengthen my leg muscles.

Every morning I got up, did all the treadmill and snow-walking-equipment exercises before my children got up. I had to push myself. I was always incredibly tired, which was probably caused by a cascading set of illnesses, such as the anemia and thyroid dysfunction. They are both autoimmune illnesses and I am convinced that the root cause of most illnesses is low sun exposure and therefore low D levels. You can read more on this on Vitamin D Wiki. It is a great site to do your own research. www.vitamindwiki.com

Looking at my esophageal illness, I researched that the esophagus cells are much like bone, cartilage and tendon cells. Bones, cartilage, and tendon cells need D to move the calcium to them and mineralize. That is why the esophagus deteriorates when D hormone levels are low. At least that is my theory for what happened to me. The reality of this piece of the puzzle is with me every day.

My conclusion and theory, based on the literature, is that once bone and cartilage have been damaged from low D levels for too long it is permanent. I know my bones have deteriorated permanently. And it is reasonable to conclude that if esophageal cells are similar to bones, cartilage, and tendon cells, that I have a permanently damaged esophagus from low D. While supplementing with D3, based on my weight, has significantly (about 98-100%) improved my laryngopharyngeal reflux, it is reasonable to conclude, as well, that my osteoarthritis of the knees is a permanent deterioration of my bones. I do feel though that having stopped the progression of osteoarthritis with D3 is saving me in the future from even further progression of the illness. Perhaps even saving me from progressing to rheumatoid arthritis like my beloved mother Demis.

It is unacceptable for babies, children, young people, and adults to suffer the wrenching consequences of preventable illnesses. The implications of low D for the populations of the planet sometimes overwhelms me because I was one of those patients who had the intractable spiral of inescapable pain. It is simply unconscionable to allow information on this common deficiency not to be part of public health education and policy and part of health prevention practices by our doctors.

I had melanoma of the foot some years back on an area of the skin where the sun rarely hits. The literature seems to imply from D scientists that melanoma is higher in people who don't get enough sunshine due to higher latitudes on the planet and having low D levels.

I had two C sections. I have a hunch from all the literature that low D scores may have significant implications on pelvis bones and ease of birthing. Not to mention the severe anemia I had during each pregnancies. The root cause: low D is suspect in my opinion.

When I was getting prepped for the fundoplication surgery, the nurse, while looking for a spot on my back to do a needle insert, asked me whether I had scoliosis. I suspect my backbone shows signs of negative bone changes.

In the early 1970s in my 20s, I suffered from pain in the right gland of my neck for five years. The ENT said he couldn't find anything wrong with me. I had a tonsillectomy at age 24 to see if that would elevate the problem. The ENT said the tissue on the tonsils showed it was not the cause of gland aching. He added that my gland in my throat was enlarged to about the size of a lemon. I suspect low levels of D in most, if not all, of these issues.

In the past decade, I have had two severe bouts of plantar fasciitis. I have a theory that the tearing of tendons that causes plantar fasciitis may indicate low D. The tendon cells are similar to bone cells and may be impacted by low D levels.

It is impossible not to ask: could the damage be permanent?

If I keep my D levels hovering at 80 ng/ml, I am free of LPR for the most part. I have had a near complete recovery in the summer, and from September through April of each year LPR returns in varying degrees – perhaps as much as five percent.

From my personal experimentation, the sun rays below the 31st latitude consistently makes my winter bit of LPR disappear completely, when I can get down below the 31st latitude.

I feel so lucky to have connected the dots and the mystery of not only what caused my current illnesses, but a lifetime of illnesses. While most of my opinions are based on the body of research I have personally studied, there is nothing that definitively states what I have pieced together for LPR. They are my conclusions and theories as a patient.

I also have a personal theory from my throat studies that all of us have a bit of acid vapor going up the throat, and the upper esophageal sphincter (UES) is supposed to close off that acid vapor that floats up from the stomach. I've pieced together from the literature that the throat is made of only one thin layer of tissue, and when the acid vapor burns through that thin throat layer, it hits the nerves that run up into the head and down the arms and legs. The vapor can even rise into the nasal cavity and down into the lungs. When this happens, the diagnosis is often asthma or allergies. I've read that autopsies have found stomach acid in people's ears. That is why I theorize D levels are essential in keeping the esophagus sphincters with "muscle twitch".

Most people complaining of acid reflux are prescribed PPIs to shut down acid production in their stomach. This can result in numerous dangerous side effects or at least it did in me. The acid of the stomach is important in the breakdown and cell uptake of nutrients. It is also thought that K1, K2, B12 and good gut microbes are adversely affected by taking PPIs. That is why sunshine and D levels are essential to maintaining muscle tone (known as muscle twitch) so that we do not begin the deterioration that medications cause.

The acid of the stomach is 50 percent of the immune system and that acid is crucial to health because it kills off viruses and bacteria that fall into your body from your nose, ears, and mouth. The acid also helps digest food and allows the cells to take up nutrients. When one's acid pumps are shut down with PPI medication, so is nutrient up take. One slowly with time on PPIs deteriorates because one is not taking up as well the nutrients in the food that is eaten through ones gastro system. When the doctor put me on proton pump inhibitors (PPIs), my legs got weak and six weeks later I developed pneumonia that would not go away until I stopped the PPIs. This explains why I got so sick on proton pump inhibitors.

Whenever I am reading a magazine or watching television, I keep a writing tablet and pencil next to me. Every time I see a new medication for any kind for illness, I write down the illness and later look it up on the internet to see if there is any connection to vitamin D. In every instance so far, all the literature points toward the possibility of low levels of D for just about everything I have researched. I am surprised by this. It is surprising what science already knows, but is not implemented in our everyday medical preventive care. And it causes a cascading list of health issues, causing medications to be prescribed as we deteriorate slowly.

One day I researched "vitamin D and breast cancer." I was shocked to learn that low D increases the odds of this devastating illness. I've queried different larger issues such as: mortality, autoimmune illnesses, heart disease, cancer of all types, diabetes, and neurological illnesses etc. There is very little that is not directly caused by low D levels.

In my readings, I've read that when a mother carries a child in utero genes can be turned off in the fetus when D levels are low. That Asperger's illness is implicated in low D levels. I was surprised to learn that if one is low in D, one is at higher risk of developing a long list of illnesses. I read that couples that are having trouble conceiving a baby, from what I have research it is worth trying to get D levels into the 40-60 ng/ml for both men and women.

I sometimes wonder if that is why children who develop severe illness after immunizations may have an immune system that is in bad need of higher D levels. I think about the military service personnel that develop depression after returning from war. Could they benefit from having their D levels increased? After all they probably went to war with low D levels and with all the gear they wear, it stands to reason they are not making vitamin D on their torso. Could it be as simple as a vitamin deficiency for a great percentage of our veterans?

Could getting vitamin D scores higher help all these health issues? My study of vitamin D has caused me to question most of my preventive healthcare thus far. I have come away from my six plus years of studying low D levels and feel that it is imperative that we address this missing piece to our prevention of illness and preventive medicine. The range of things that D does in our body is so far reaching, it will be a long time before scientists fully understand the implications to our short and long term health when we are chronically low on vitamin D throughout our lives.

Science writers like Dr. Oliver Gillie of the UK, my favorite science writer, has also written numerous important papers that I consider my go-to D file. I actually keep his articles front and center when I go back to review things I have learned. Dr. Gillie is worth looking up and reading all his work and seeing his lectures on YouTube. I just can't thank him enough for all the papers he has authored and shared with the world. And he did all of his work without pay and alone.

I used to suffer from insomnia. According to the theory of Texas neurologist, Dr. Stasha Gominak of Texas, low levels of vitamin D can prevent a person from getting to the stage of "paralyzing sleep," where the body's repair processes take place. In fact, Dr. Gominak's interest in sleep disorders has led her to theorize that D is critical to health in many ways.

Another wonderful online resource is Grassroots Health (grassrootshealth.net), which is comprised of international scientists that study and promote awareness of the need for appropriate levels of vitamin D. The website includes a chart linking various illnesses with vitamin D deficiency and new research. Stunning is all I can say when one fully realizes the implications.

And there are many more. We only need to do our own research. The science is there, but our doctors are either not trained in medical school about this or it is just missing as part of preventive medicine. It is a health crisis of enormous proportions and we as patients can do something about.

CHAPTER 13

MY OBSERVATIONS

I am keenly aware that my journey through illness and my recovery, and observations are merely anecdotal. They are only my personal opinions and theories as a patient for all the health issues I had throughout my lifetime and those of my family and friends. But if what I have managed to figure out as a patient from research is correct, then we have the answers to so many illnesses that plague us in modern times.

In this final chapter I would like to share a few experiences with people I know that have caused me to look at hormone D in a broader perspective and made me think that I might have something to share from personal experience.

The first experience happened around the end of October 2011, about two months after I started my own D treatment. At that time I was thinking of D only in terms of my own health. About that time, a friend's mother, then age 87, had to go to the emergency room of her local hospital by ambulance. She was admitted and in the hospital for three weeks.

During the first week she was so weak, she could not raise her arms. She had no appetite. She was unable to sit up. Her adult children gathered in her hospital room. They were all worried. My friend told me how shocked they were when the attending physician said to the elderly lady: "Why did you come to the ER? You are dying. You should have just stayed home and died. There is nothing more we can do for you. Go home and die at home." He turned to the oldest sibling and urged him to sign off on his mother. There would only be palliative care from then on.

When I heard about this, I paused thinking about all the things I had been reading about Vitamin D. The woman had been retired for 27 years. She never went outside. And she lived at a latitude where it is hard to obtain vitamin D from the sun.

I could not stop myself. I said, "Don't sign anything. Tell the doctor you want your mom off as many medications as possible. Have her D levels taken immediately." It was done. Her D levels were very low. She was then given supplements of D3. Her appetite picked up slowly. After several weeks, she was released from hospital. I told the family to obtain home care and get her outside when the sun was high. To our amazement, the woman was able to get around with a walking aid, and eventually within three months only needed a simple walking cane.

My friends said they would love to parade their mother in front of the doctor of "death" so that he could see how well the "dying" patient was doing. We all feel quite sure the D3 has helped her make a remarkable recovery. And to put a final good note on this story, my friend told me six months later that the mother, who had been losing her hair for ten years, had grown a full head of hair!

I think low D levels causes a slow progressive slide into poor health, decade after decade, which cascades into illness and causes doctors to put patients on medications that worsen the situation. We know none of us will live forever, but how wonderful to feel as good as one can for as long as one can. At the time of this writing in 2017, the woman is 93 years old and going strong. We are all amazed. No one more so than me.

My next story is about a friend who came for a visit. He stayed overnight, and when he got up in the morning, my husband and I were sipping our coffee in the living room. I asked our guest whether he had slept well. "Not so good," he said. I wondered whether the guest's room was chilly, or whether the bed was uncomfortable. "No," he said, "I just can't sleep. I've been taking sleeping pills for 10 years and can't sleep. They are not working anymore." I paused, thinking where have I read this before!? I asked him if he had other symptoms. He said that in addition to not being able to sleep even with sleeping pills, he suffered from chronic fatigue. To get some exercise, he tried to walk on a treadmill, but was unable to do so for more than three minutes.

I looked at my husband and back at our friend, and I thought, could it be low D? Something clicked inside my mind, based on all the research I had been doing. "Would you trust me on this?" I asked. "Go get your vitamin D level checked as soon as you go back home. Promise me you will?" He said he would.

Three days later, our guest phoned and asked to speak to me. Our friend said to me, "My doctor wanted to know how did I know to ask for a D test?! I told him that you told me to. My test came back, and my doctor said my D level is only 11 ng/mL, and that I'm very sick. My doctor is putting me on 50,000 IU of D right away."

When I looked up the vitamin D sleep connection, I found that there is a theory that D affects the ability to fall asleep and stay asleep. And that sleep helps our nighttime hormone come out to do its work of healing our body. My hunch listening to our friend turned out correct. Our friend is doing dramatically better since he got on D. He often thanks me for getting him to the doctor to be tested. I feel I'm fortunate that I continue to study and can begin to recognize that my family and friends probably have very low D levels. In fact most people I run across everyday have low D levels. They all have different ailments, but in each instance I research their illness and the root cause seems to be decades of low D levels.

What I've gleaned from research is that the effects of D levels are so far-reaching, scientists still have not discovered all that this hormone does in our bodies. But for my thinking, it stands to reason, we are not roaming the forests anymore. In modern society we are inside quite a bit and it is causing skyrocketing illness. And a great many of us live above the 31st latitude, which predisposes us to greater incidence of all types of illnesses.

My research indicates that sunshine is the best way to get hormone D, and taking supplements should be secondary. There is something about the direct sunshine that cannot be duplicated in the D3. I feel it in my own experimentation with myself. I've read recently that one of the newer discoveries about sunshine is that the sun exposure produces not only D, but also cholesterol on the skin and nitric oxide. It sounds as though cholesterol sulfate is very important for all cells, especially red blood cells. And nitric oxide lowers blood pressure. It is pretty well accepted science that blood pressure rises in the winter above the 31st latitude. Could that have some relationship to anemia, an autoimmune illness I suffered from all my life?

I also wonder often wonder why a doctor would not be curious about how and why D worked for me. I am hoping that my firsthand experience will find its way to the Institutes of Medicine and our public health leaders, who will consider the suffering of so many patients and the economic financial drain on people and our national treasury because of low D levels since utero. I hope that our Institute of Medicine will listen to the scientists who are doing research in this area. The money alone that could be saved by citizens, and governments worldwide would be stunning.

My bones are arthritic from too many decades of low D levels. The cartilage is destroyed. None of my doctors ever thought of low D. I remember going in to see my primary in the early 2000s, bringing an article that recommended asking for a bone sonogram to check for osteomalacia. My doctor really didn't see the need to do it, but because I insisted she ordered the test.

I had osteomalacia she said and I could take some calcium, but I remember she was not concerned about it. And no doctor connected it with my thyroid illness, or my chronic anemia, chronic colds and flus that plagued me all my life, fatigue, melanoma and difficulty during my pregnancies and so on. I believe sincerely that all my illnesses are connected to low D. In fact I'm as sure about it as one can be.

It is too late for my bones and my muscle "twitch". They have permanent damage. But D3 and direct sunshine on the whole torso have given me my quality of life back. I'm not "cured", but I am in a "remission" of sorts, for lack of a better word. I have probably stopped the progression of arthritis to other more serious bone issues. I'm due soon for knees replacements. My orthopedic surgeon told me in 2013 that I was too young for a knee replacement. A lifetime of low D levels causes damage to the bones, muscles, cartilage, tendons and all biological systems of the human body. It is now 2018 and with D3 and omega 3's I have held off pain and knee replacements. For how long remains to be seen.

My pregnancies were from hell. I was told early through both pregnancies that I would be put in the hospital for the duration of my pregnancies due to the severity of my anemia. I had to eat liver several times a day to avoid the hospital. Anemia is thought to be an autoimmune illness (as is thyroid illness, heart disease and so many other illnesses). My pregnancies exasperated the problem. I look back now and realize that there is a link to low D levels. Additionally my babies had severe colic, which I have a theory is caused by low D.

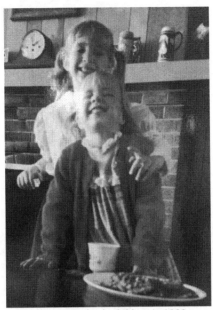

Figure 8 Author's children in 1982.

My first child not only suffered through severe colic, but she also had severe ear infections. By the time she was 20 months old in 1980, she had been on thirteen bottles of antibiotics nonstop since she was ten months old and was near death when she required an emergency ear surgery for an ear infection that had gone out of control. The surgery could not be performed for three days as her fever was so high they had to hope they could bring it down with intravenous antibiotics before they could go in and see how far the infection had traveled. The doctor was incredulous that the infection did not break through the inner ear membrane to the brain. Her ears drained very dark green ooze for four days after surgery. I look back and wonder if low D was the root cause of all this illness in her.

From 1984-1988 my children suffered with nonstop illnesses (colds that would go away and come back a week later) from about three to seven years of age. The doctors were at a loss as to what was causing it. They blamed it on allergies. My children went through a lot as we worked with the doctor to eliminate foods that they thought could be causing it. I now wonder if it was low D levels.

One day when writing this book and discussing it with my youngest daughter, who was my rock and support during my severe illness, I asked her on the spur of the moment, "Honey, how did you know that my illness was not caused by stress like the doctors said?" She looked at me and said, "Mama, I know you. Growing up you never complained about anything even when you were sick, so I knew without a doubt there was something really wrong with you." I cannot say how much that meant to me to hear that from my daughter.

I hope that my readers will be able to address evolutionary needs much sooner than I did. I hope mothers and fathers before they have children get their US D scores up to the Grassroots recommendation of 40-60 ng/mL to give their baby the best chance at a healthy start in life (Canada and the UK have a different D scoring system).

In conclusion, I believe my LPR is a permanent chronic condition I will always have to monitor by myself for the rest of my life. Although, it is in a "remission" of sorts for lack of a better word, I believe the long term effects of low D on the esophagus and muscles of the throat caused my LPR and other illnesses. And maybe even the severe sleep apnea I have. One can imagine from just reading the literature on D, what other damage has been done to other organs, gene and cell function. It is a consequence of my decades (since utero) of low D levels. And it is an irony that a D test cost so much that I can't afford it at my healthcare provider currently. It should be free because a D lab test should be a free test for everyone in the world. It is one of the most basic health preventive measures that can be done on any patient worldwide.

We all want to live as long as we can with the best quality of health we can have. Adequate vitamin D levels is fundamental to that goal. But it will take citizens to research and start demanding that D levels be part of preventive healthcare.

We cannot afford to stand by and wait for the medical community to implement this for us. Let us globally insist that our medical professionals do D testing as part of preventive care and that they guide and educate the public with public health messages to keep our D levels high enough. D tests should be done not just at hospital labs, but should be done wherever it can be set up so that it is convenient for the public to get tested. Let us make this a top medical priority of our time.

It took me six months after discovering D to find out that that there are so many scientists working on getting the word out on vitamin D. I will put a few of my most favorite web links here that will help you start your own research:

The Health Research Forum from the UK has seven reports at this time that have far reaching implications for our worldwide   health   --
www.healthresearchforum.org.uk/reports.html

The scientist/writer Oliver Gillie's papers are an eye opening view into what is already known about Vitamin D. Why do I love reading his papers on the subject? They are so interesting. Dr. Gillie's work is phenomenal. They are my bible on vitamin D3 and sunshine!

Vitamin D Wiki: www.vitamindwiki.com/VitaminDWiki

Disease Incidence Prevention Chart from Grassroots Health website: www.grassrootshealth.net. This chart is worth keeping on your refrigerator!

Disease Incidence Prevention Chart from Grassroots Health website for pregnancy and young children: www.grassrootshealth.net

Grassroots Health: www.grassrootshealth.net

This site is worth sharing with everyone you love and worth discussing with your family. Phenomenal site. The work that the Vitamin D scientists do every day deserves our gratitude for their courage to get the word out.

YouTube Video Dr. Cedric Garland, UCSD TV Vitamin D and Sunlight for Cancer Prevention 2014: www.ucsd.tv

Vitamin D for Health A Global Perspective by Arash Hossein-Nezhad, MD, PHD and Michael Holick, PHD, MD on the Mayo Clinic's website: www.mayoclinicproceedings.org

Vitamin D and Human Skeletal Muscle by B. Hamilton: www.ncbi.nlm.nih.gov

Vitamin D and the Digestive System by W. Stumpf www.unc.edu

Dr. Stasha Gominak: www.drgominak.com

Dr. Gominak ties together her observations and shares her theories.

There are thousands of papers, articles, lectures, videos worth reading and reviewing for most of the illnesses we as a global population suffer from. You will soon find that you will be enthralled by what science already knows about sunshine and high enough D scores. It will be an illumination and great personal discovery for you and the people you love. It will answer why our illnesses have gotten so much worse in modern times.

I wish my readers a long and good life.

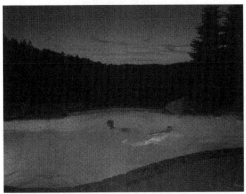

Figure 9 Author watching her grandchildren in the pool during her devastating illness.

I almost lost everything…

Because of Vitamin D, I'm still here to enjoy watching my grandchildren.

My gratitude goes to all the D scientists around the world whose work has confirmed what I accidently discovered in my desperate search for answers.

My theory is that the oldest hormone in our evolution: the lack of high enough levels of master Hormone D is the root cause for 50-75% of most illnesses.

We are only at the beginning of understanding the far reaching implications of being removed from the sunshine and moving up the latitude of the planet as a species.

I wish my readers the best in their personal journey of discovery, recovery and triumph over a wide range of illnesses.

ABOUT THE AUTHOR

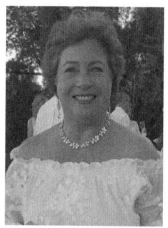

Figure 10 September 2016

Eva Cardoza King was born and raised in San Francisco, California, attending local schools: St. Anthony and Immaculate Conception Academy (ICA). She graduated with a BA in Behavioral Science from the University of Maine at Presque Isle, Maine, and has a Master's in Public Administration from the Notre Dame University in Belmont, California.

Eva is married, has two grown daughters and two grandchildren, and lives in the Foothills of Northern California.

Eva shares her experience with devastating illnesses and how she connected the dots through personal research, and successfully diagnosed and treated herself. She remains in "remission" of all illnesses at this time.

The author believes that 50-70% of all illnesses point directly to an inexpensive substance that is lacking in most of our modern lives.

Made in the USA
San Bernardino, CA
04 March 2019